Mediterranean Diet Coo

Easy and Flavorful Recipes to Maintain a Healthy Lifestyle with 4-Week Weight Loss Meal Plan

Kendall Cobb

Table of Contents

BREAKFAST

For more tips go to: Growthshape.com/health

01. Salmon and Bulgur Salad

Preparation time: 25 minutes

Cooking time: 10 minutes

Servings:4

Ingredients:

- 1 pound salmon fillet, skinless and boneless
- 1 tablespoon olive oil
- 1 cup bulgur
- 1 cup parsley, chopped
- ¼ cup mint, chopped
- 3 tablespoons lemon juice
- 1 red onion, sliced
- Salt and black pepper to the taste
- 2 cup hot water

Directions:

- Heat up a pan with half of the oil over medium heat, add the salmon, some salt and pepper, cook for 5 minutes on each side, cool down, flake and put in a salad bowl.
- In another bowl, mix the bulgur with hot water, cover, leave aside for 25 minutes, drain and transfer to the bowl with the salmon.
- Add the rest of the ingredients, toss and serve for breakfast.

Nutrition Values: calories 321, fat 11.3, fiber 7.9, carbs 30.8, protein 27.6

02. Herbed Quinoa and Asparagus

Preparation time: 10 minutes

Cooking time: 0 minutes

Servings:4

Ingredients:

- 3 cups asparagus, steamed and roughly chopped
- 1 tablespoon olive oil
- 3 tablespoons balsamic vinegar
- 1 and ¾ cups quinoa, cooked
- 2 teaspoons mustard
- Salt and black pepper to the taste
- 5 ounces baby spinach
- ½ cup parsley, chopped
- 1 tablespoon thyme, chopped
- 1 tablespoon tarragon, chopped

Directions:

1. In a salad bowl, combine the asparagus with the quinoa, spinach and the rest of the ingredients, toss and keep in the fridge for 10 minutes before serving for breakfast.

Nutrition Values:calories 323, fat 11.3, fiber 3.4, carbs 16.4, protein 10

03. Lettuce and Strawberry Salad

Preparation time: 5 minutes

Cooking time: 0 minutes

Servings:6

Ingredients:

- 1 avocado, peeled, pitted and mashed
- 2 tablespoons almond milk
- 1 tablespoon poppy seeds
- 4 cups romaine lettuce leaves, torn
- 1 tablespoon balsamic vinegar
- 1 cup strawberries, sliced
- 2 tablespoons almonds, toasted and chopped

Directions:

1. In a bowl, mix the avocado with the lettuce and the rest of the ingredients, toss and serve for breakfast,

Nutrition Values: calories 145, fat 1.9, fiber 1.2, carbs 3.6, protein 2.3

04. Ham Cups

Preparation time: 15 minutes

Cooking time: 5 minutes

Servings: 6

Ingredients:

- 10 oz. ham, sliced
- 6 eggs, beaten
- 5 oz. Cheddar cheese, shredded
- 1 tablespoon olive oil
- 1 tablespoon fresh parsley, chopped

Directions:

2. Wipe the muffin molds with the olive oil.
3. Place the sliced ham in the muffin molds in the shape of the cups.
4. Pour the beaten eggs over the ham.
5. Sprinkle the eggs with the chopped parsley and shredded cheese.
6. Place the molds on a trivet.
7. Pour 1 cup of water into the instant pot bowl.
8. Place the trivet in the instant pot.
9. Close the lid and cook the meal for 5 minutes on High pressure.
10. When the meal is cooked, do a natural pressure release and serve the breakfast!

Nutrition Values:calories 252, fat 18.2, fiber 0.6, carbs 2.5, protein 19.3

SEAFOOD

05. Raw Spanish Mackerel in Lime and Coconut Cream

Preparation time: 8 hours

Servings: 2

Ingredients:

- Spanish mackerel-1lb
- Red onion, diced-1tablespoon
- Lime juice-1cup
- Cucumber, -2
- Spring onion, diced-1teaspoon
- Lime juice-1teaspoon
- Coconut cream-1 1/2cup
- Red chili -1
- Tomato, diced-1cup
- Salt to taste

Directions:

1. Peel the cucumber. Discard the seeds and dice them.
2. Chop the red chili and discard the seeds.
3. Cut the fish into small pieces.
4. In a bowl add the lime juice. Soak the fish in it for 4 hours.
5. Drain and transfer to a bowl.
6. Add the tomato, salt, red chili, coconut cream, lime juice, spring onion, cucumber,

and red onion.

7. Mix well and refrigerate for about 4 hours or longer.

8. Serve cold.

06. Easy Pan Fried Fish

Preparation time: 30 minutes

Ingredients:

- ounce fish fillets cod, halibut, Mahi, or any firm white fish
- medium sliced red pepper
- tbsps. Olive oil
- tsp. dried basil
- ½ large onion: sliced
- large garlic cloves: chopped
- 1/3 cup pitted Kalamata olives
- ¼ cup chicken stock
- ½ cup halved cherry tomatoes
- ¼ cup white wine
- Salt and pepper to taste
- Garnish: feta, fresh parsley or chopped basil as desired

Directions:

1. Dry fish with a paper towel to remove moisture then sprinkle with salt and pepper.
2. Cut vegetables into slices and put away.
3. Heat non-stick frying pan or skillet to medium heat, add olive oil and leave to get hot for 30 seconds or until hot.
4. Put fish onto the pan and let it sear for 3 to 4 minutes on each side. Do not try moving the fish as it sears. When the fish is not stuck to the pan, it is ready to be flipped. Remove the fish from the pan and put aside.
5. Put onions and sliced red pepper onto the pan and let cook for 2 to 3 minutes or

until it is slightly soft then add tomatoes and garlic. Season the mixture with pepper and salt.

6. Scrape vegetables stuck to the pan and add white wine, chicken stock, and basil.

7. Add fish to pan and cook for 3 to 4 minutes until fish breaks apart easily.

8. Put Kalamata olives into the pan and allow to heat slightly.

9. Serve with fresh basil, fresh parsley, and lemon wedges or a sprinkle of feta.

07. Caper Garnished Baked Fish and Tomatoes

Preparation time: 35 minutes

Servings: 6

Ingredients:

- 2 large tomatoes: diced or quality canned tomatoes
- 1/3 cup extra virgin oil
- 10 garlic cloves: chopped
- small red onion: finely chopped
- tsp. Organic ground cumin
- ½ tsp. cayenne pepper (optional)
- tsp. All natural sweet Spanish paprika
- ½ tsp. organic ground coriander
- ½ tbsp. capers
- 1/3 cup golden raisins
- ½ juiced lemon or more (as preferred)
- whole lemon zest
- Fresh parsley or mint
- ½ Ib. Whitefish fillets such as halibut or cod
- Salt and pepper

Directions:

1. Capers and tomato sauce.
2. Heat olive oil in a medium saucepan over medium-high heat and add onions. Cook for 3 minutes, tossing regularly, until golden. Add tomatoes, spices, garlic and a pinch of salt and pepper, capers and raisins. Bring mixture to a boil and turn the heat

down to medium-low and simmer for 15 minutes.

3. Heat oven to 400°F.

4. Dry fish with a paper towel to remove moisture then season on both sides with salt and pepper.

5. In a 9 ½ x 13 inches baking dish, pour half of the cooked tomato sauce and layer the fish on top to cover the sauce. Add lemon zest and juice and then top with the remaining tomato sauce.

6. Bake in the oven for 15 to 18 minutes or until the fish is cooked through or breaks easily. Make sure not to overcook.

7. Remove from the oven and garnish with mint or fresh parsley.

8. Serve immediately with Greek potatoes, Lebanese rice or Mediterranean grilled zucchini.

08. Fried Tilapia with Vegetables and Rice

Preparation time: 20 minutes

Servings: 4

Ingredients:

- tbsp. Butter
- tbsps. Capers
- tsp. Garlic: crushed
- cup baby spinach: densely packed; chopped
- 1/3 cup sun-dried tomatoes: chopped
- Ib. Tilapia or other white fish
- 12 oz. jar, Aldi artichoke salad or another alternative

Directions:

1. Thaw the fish if it is frozen and pat dry with paper towel to remove moisture.
2. In a sauté pan, melt butter under medium-high heat.
3. Put fish in sauté pan and allow to brown on both sides for 2 minutes.
4. Add vegetables, tomatoes, and other Ingredients: and cook over medium heat for 5-10 minutes.
5. Serve with rice, cauliflower rice or eat as it is.

09. Baked Tilapia Fillets

Preparation time: 25 minutes.Serves 4.

Ingredients:

- tsp. Olive oil
- tbsp. Bitter
- Ib. Tilapia fillets (8 fillets)
- garlic cloves: minced
- shallots: finely chopped
- ½ tsp. Paprika
- ½ tsp. Ground cumin
- ¼ cup fresh dill: finely chopped
- lemon: juiced
- ¼ cup capers
- Salt and pepper

Directions:

1. Heat oven to 375°.
2. Line a rimmed baking sheet with foil or parchment paper and spray with cooking spray then spread fish on it
3. Mix salt, pepper, cumin and paprika in a small bowl and season the fish, on both sides, with the mixture.
4. In another bowl, mix the melted butter, olive oil, shallots, garlic, and lemon juice. Brush the mixture over the fish and top with capers.
5. Bake for 10-15 minutes in the oven. Avoid overcooking it.
6. Remove and serve topped with fresh dill.

10. Lemony Orzo pasta with Baked Fish Fillets.

Preparation time: 30 minutes

Servings: 4

Ingredients:

- Sauce
- tsp. Garlic: minced
- shallots: minced
- tbsp. Olive oil
- ½ to 1 tsp. Red pepper: crushed
- tsp. dried anise seed
- tsp. Anchovy paste
- tbsp. Fresh oregano leaves: chopped or 1 tsp. Dried oregano
- tbsps. Capers: rinsed and drained
- tbsps. Olive tapenade recipe
- 1/5 ounces can crushed tomatoes
- Fish
- 16-24 oz. firm, white fish fillets: rinsed and patted dry
- Italian parsley
- 1-ounce feta cheese: crumbled
- Lemony orzo
- shallot: minced
- cups vegetable/ chicken stock: cooking on low heat
- Olive oil

- lemon: zest and juice

Directions:

1. Preheat oven to 400°.
2. Heat olive oil in sauté pan on medium heat.
3. Add shallots, crushed pepper, anchovy paste, and garlic. Sauté until mixture is fragrant and shallots are nearly translucent.
4. Mix in anise seed and oregano leaves and sauté for 1 minute.
5. Add Tapenade, tomatoes, capers and fresh oregano.
6. Reduce heat and let it simmer for 5 minutes.

Fish

7. Choose a medium sized pan so that fillets will be cozy but not crowded.
8. Put 2/3 of the tomato sauce in the pan and spread evenly. Arrange fish in a single layer, leave it if it extends over another.
9. Spread remaining sauce over the fish and the center of the pan.
10. Please put it in the oven and cook for 5-10 minutes until the fish starts to look cloudy or opaque.
11. Remove the fish and sprinkle with crumbled feta then return to the oven for another 5 minutes. Avoid overcooking.
12. Remove from the oven.
13. Tilapia and flounder fillet, as used in this recipe, requires a cooking time of 10-15 minutes in a convection oven and 12-18 minutes in a standard oven. The thickness of the fillets determines the cooking time.

Lemony Orzo

14. Drizzle some olive oil and add shallots to a medium saucepan on medium-high heat.
15. Sauté until shallots are nearly translucent and mix in the orzo.
16. Zest lemon and set aside.

17. Squeeze juice without seeds over the orzo and stir in thoroughly.

18. Add hot broth to the pan slowly (a ladle at a time) and allow the orzo to absorb it without getting soft then stir in zest.

19. Serve each plate with a fish fillet and some sauce from the pan (if necessary) with the lemony orzo and garnish with chopped Italian parsley.

POULTRY

11. Chicken and Ginger Cucumbers Mix

Preparation time: 10 minutes

Cooking time: 20 minutes

Servings:4

Ingredients:

- 4 chicken breasts, boneless, skinless and cubed
- 2 cucumbers, cubed
- Salt and black pepper to the taste
- tablespoon ginger, grated
- tablespoon garlic, minced
- tablespoons balsamic vinegar
- tablespoons olive oil
- ¼ teaspoon chili paste
- ½ cup chicken stock
- ½ tablespoon lime juice
- tablespoon chives, chopped

Directions:

1. Heat up a pan with the oil over medium-high heat, add the chicken and brown for 3 minutes on each side.
2. Add the cucumbers, salt, pepper and the rest of the ingredients except the chives, bring to a simmer and cook over medium heat for 15 minutes.

3. Divide the mix between plates and serve with the chives sprinkled on top.

Nutrition Values:calories 288, fat 9.5, fiber 12.1, carbs 25.6, protein 28.6

12. Turmeric Chicken and Eggplant Mix

Preparation time: 10 minutes

Cooking time: 30 minutes

Servings:4

Ingredients:

- 2 cups eggplant, cubed
- Salt and black pepper to the taste
- 2 tablespoons olive oil
- cup yellow onion, chopped
- tablespoons garlic, minced
- tablespoons hot paprika
- teaspoon turmeric powder
- and ½ tablespoons oregano, chopped
- cup chicken stock
- pound chicken breast, skinless, boneless and cubed
- cup half and half
- tablespoon lemon juice

Directions:

1. Heat up a pan with the oil over medium-high heat, add the chicken and brown for 4 minutes on each side.
2. Add the eggplant, onion and garlic and sauté for 5 minutes more.
3. Add the rest of the ingredients, bring to a simmer and cook over medium heat for 16 minutes.
4. Divide the mix between plates and serve.

Nutrition Values:calories 392, fat 11.6, fiber 8.3, carbs 21.1, protein 24.2

13. Tomato Chicken and Lentils

Preparation time: 10 minutes

Cooking time: 1 hour

Servings:8

Ingredients:

- 2 tablespoons olive oil
- 2 celery stalks, chopped
- red onion, chopped
- tablespoons tomato paste
- garlic cloves, chopped
- ½ cup chicken stock
- 2 cups French lentils
- pound chicken thighs, boneless and skinless
- Salt and black pepper to the taste
- tablespoon cilantro, chopped

Directions:

1. Heat up a Dutch oven with the oil over medium-high heat, add the onion and the garlic and sauté for 2 minutes.
2. Add the chicken and brown for 3 minutes on each side.
3. Add the rest of the ingredients except the cilantro, bring to a simmer and cook over medium-low heat for 45 minutes.
4. Add the cilantro, stir, divide the mix into bowls and serve.

Nutrition Values:calories 249, fat 9.7, fiber 11.9, carbs 25.3, protein 24.3

14. Turkey, Leeks and Carrots

Preparation time: 10 minutes

Cooking time: 1 hour

Servings:4

Ingredients:

- big turkey breast, skinless, boneless and cubed
- tablespoons avocado oil
- Salt and black pepper to the taste
- 1 tablespoon sweet paprika
- ½ cup chicken stock
- 1 leek, sliced
- 1 carrot, sliced
- 1 yellow onion, chopped
- 1 tablespoon lemon juice
- 1 teaspoon cumin, ground
- 1 tablespoon basil, chopped

Directions:

1. Heat up a pan with the oil over medium-high heat, add the turkey and brown for 4 minutes on each side.
2. Add the leeks, carrot and the onion and sauté everything for 5 minutes more.
3. Add the rest of the ingredients, bring to a simmer and cook over medium heat for 40 minutes.
4. Divide the mix between plates and serve.

Nutrition Values:calories 249, fat 10.7, fiber 11.9, carbs 22.3, protein 17.3

MEAT

For more tips go to: Growthshape.com/health

15. Delightful Citrus Sautéed Spinach

Servings: 4

Preparationtime: 5 minutes

Cooking time: 5 minutes

Ingredients:

- 1 teaspoon orange zest
- 1/2 teaspoon sea salt
- 1/4 cup orange juice
- 1/8 teaspoon black pepper
- 2 tablespoons olive oil
- 4 cups fresh spinach

Directions:

1. In a large pan over medium-high heat heat the olive oil until it simmers.
2. mix spinach and orange zest. Cook for about 3 minutes stirring occasionally until the spinach browned.
3. mix the orange juice sea salt and pepper. Cook for 2 minutes stirring occasionally. Serve hot.

16. Healthy Masked Cauliflower

Servings: 4

Preparationtime: 10 minutes

Cooking time: 15 minutes

Ingredients:

- 1/2 teaspoon sea salt
- 1/4 cup (2 ounces) Parmesan cheese
- 1/4 cup skimmed milk
- 1/8 teaspoon black pepper
- 2 tablespoons butter
- 2 tablespoons olive oil
- 4 cups cauliflower florets

Directions:

1. In a vast bowl over medium heat cover the cauliflower with water and bring it a boil. lessen the heat to medium cover and simmer for 10 minutes until cauliflower is soft.

2. Drain cauliflower and return it to pot. mix milk cheese butter olive oil sea salt and pepper. Using a potato masher mash until smooth.

MAIN DISH

17. Traditional Bolognese Sauce

Preparation Time: 35 minutes

Servings: 6

Nutrition Values: Calories 318, Fat: 20g; Net Carbs: 5.9g; Protein: 26g

Ingredients

- 1 onion, chopped
- 1½ pounds ground beef
- 2 garlic cloves, minced
- 1 tsp marjoram
- 1 tsp rosemary
- 4 tomatoes, chopped
- 1 tbsp olive oil

Directions

1. Heat olive oil in a saucepan over medium heat. Add onion and garlic and cook for 3 minutes. Add beef and cook until browned, about 4-5 minutes. Stir in the herbs and tomatoes. Cook for 15 minutes.

18. Baked Zucchini Stuffed with Shrimp & Dill

Preparation Time: 56 minutes

Servings: 4

Nutrition Values: Calories 135, Fat 14.4g; Net Carbs 3.2g; Protein 24.6g

Ingredients

- 2 tbsp olive oil
- 20 oz medium zucchinis
- 1 lb small shrimp, peeled, deveined
- ½ onion, minced
- 2 tsp butter
- 2 tomatoes, chopped
- Salt and black pepper to taste
- 1 cup pork rinds, crushed
- 1 tbsp fresh dill, chopped

Directions

2. Trim off the top and bottom ends of the zucchinis. Lay them flat on a chopping board, and cut a ¼-inch off the top to create a boat for the stuffing. Scoop out the seeds with a spoon and set the zucchinis aside.

3. Melt the butter in a small skillet and sauté the onion and tomato for 6 minutes. Transfer the mixture to a bowl and add the shrimp, half of the pork rinds, fresh dill, salt, and pepper.

4. Combine the ingredients and stuff the zucchini boats with the mixture. Sprinkle the top of the boats with the remaining pork rinds and drizzle the olive oil over them.

5. Place on a baking sheet and bake them for 15 to 20 minutes at 350°F. The shrimp should no longer be pink by this time. Remove the zucchinis after and serve with a

tomato and mozzarella salad.

19. Garlic Chicken with Anchovy Paste

Preparation Time: 30 minutes

Servings: 2

Nutrition Values: Calories 155, Fat 13g; Net Carbs 3g; Protein 25g

Ingredients

- ½ pound chicken breast, cut into 4 pieces
- 2 tbsp olive oil
- 3 garlic cloves, crushed
- For the paste
- 1 cup black olives, pitted
- 4 anchovy fillets, rinsed
- 1 garlic clove, crushed
- Salt and black pepper, to taste
- 2 tbsp olive oil
- ¼ cup fresh basil, chopped
- 1 tbsp lemon juice

Directions

1. Using a food processor, combine the olives, salt, olive oil, basil, lemon juice, anchovy fillets, and pepper, blend well. Set a pan over medium heat and warm olive oil, stir-fry in the garlic and chicken and cook for 10 minutes. Remove to a serving plate and top with anchovy paste to serve.

20. Sardines Skillet with Zucchini Spaghetti

Preparation Time: 10 minutes

Servings: 2

Nutrition Values: Calories 355, Fat: 31g; Net Carbs: 6g; Protein: 20g

Ingredients

- 32 oz zucchini spaghetti
- 2 oz cubed pancetta
- 4 oz canned sardines, chopped
- ½ cup canned tomatoes, chopped
- 4 green olives, pitted and chopped
- 1 tbsp parsley
- 1 garlic clove, minced

Directions

1. Pour some of the sardine oil in a skillet. Add garlic and cook for 1 minute. Add pancetta and cook for 2 minutes. Stir in the tomatoes and let simmer for 5 minutes. Add zucchini spaghetti and sardines and cook for 3 minutes. Remove to a platter and scatter the green olives on top to serve.

21. Buttered Garlic Shrimp

Preparation Time: 22 minutes

Servings: 6

Nutrition Values: Calories 258, Fat 22g; Net Carbs 2g; Protein 13g

Ingredients

- 4 oz butter

- 2 lbshrimp, peeled and deveined

- Sea salt and black pepper to taste

- A pinch of red pepper flakes

- 3 garlic cloves, minced

- 3 tbsp water

- 1 lemon, zested and juiced

- 2 tbsp fresh parsley, chopped

Directions

2. Warm half of the butter in a large skillet over medium heat, season the shrimp with salt, pepper, pepper flakes, and add to the butter. Stir in the garlic and cook the shrimp for 4 minutes on both sides until pink. Remove to a bowl and set aside.

3. Put the remaining butter in the skillet; include the lemon zest, juice, and water. Cook until the butter has melted, about 1 minute. Add the shrimp and adjust the taste with salt and black pepper. Cook for 2 minutes on low heat. Serve the shrimp sprinkled with parsley.

SIDE DISH

For more tips go to: Growthshape.com/health

22. Eggplant and Bell Pepper Mix

Preparation time: 10 minutes

Cooking time: 45 minutes

Servings:4

Ingredients:

- 2 green bell peppers, cut into strips
- 2 eggplants, sliced
- 2 tablespoons tomato paste
- Salt and black pepper to the taste
- 4 garlic cloves, minced
- ¼ cup olive oil
- 1 tablespoon cilantro, chopped
- 1 tablespoon chives, chopped

Directions:

1. In a roasting pan, combine the bell peppers with the eggplants and the rest of the ingredients, introduce in the oven and cook at 380 degrees F for 45 minutes.
2. Divide the mix between plates and serve as a side dish.

Nutrition Values:calories 207, fat 13.3, fiber 10.5, carbs 23.4, protein 3.8

23. Basil and Sun-dried Tomatoes Rice

Preparation time: 10 minutes

Cooking time: 25 minutes

Servings:4

Ingredients:

- 5 cups chicken stock
- 1 yellow onion, chopped
- ounces sun dried tomatoes in olive oil, drained and chopped
- 2 cups Arborio rice
- Salt and black pepper to the taste
- 1 and ½ cup parmesan, grated
- 2 tablespoons olive oil
- ¼ cup basil leaves, chopped

Directions:

1. Heat up a pan with the oil over medium heat, add the onion and the tomatoes and sauté for 5 minutes.
2. Add the rice, stock and the rest of the ingredients except the parmesan, bring to a simmer and cook over medium heat for 20 minutes.
3. Add the parmesan, toss, divide the mix between plates and serve as a side dish.

Nutrition Values:calories 426, fat 8.4, fiber 3.2, carbs 56.3, protein 7.5

24. Dill Cucumber Salad

Preparation time: 1 hour

Cooking time: 0 minutes

Servings:8

Ingredients:

- 4 cucumbers, sliced

- 1 cup white wine vinegar

- 2 white onions, sliced

- 1 tablespoon dill, chopped

Directions:

1. In a bowl, mix the cucumber with the onions, vinegar and the dill, toss well and keep in the fridge for 1 hour before serving as a side salad.

Nutrition Values:calories 182, fat 3.5, fiber 4.5, carbs 8.5, protein 4.5

25. Herbed Cucumber and Avocado Mix

Preparation time: 10 minutes

Cooking time: 0 minutes

Servings:4

Ingredients:

- 2 cucumbers, sliced
- 2 avocados, pitted, peeled and cubed
- 1 tablespoon lemon juice
- 3 tablespoons olive oil
- 2 teaspoons balsamic vinegar
- 1 teaspoon dill, dried
- 1 tablespoon cilantro, chopped
- 1 tablespoon chives, chopped
- 1 tablespoon basil, chopped
- 1 tablespoon oregano, chopped

Directions:

1. In a bowl, mix the cucumbers with the avocados with the rest of the ingredients, toss and serve as a side dish.

Nutrition Values:calories 343, fat 9.6, fiber 2.5, carbs 16.5, protein 7.4

26. Basil Bell Peppers and Cucumber Mix

Preparation time: 5 minutes

Cooking time: 0 minutes

Servings:6

Ingredients:

- 1 red bell pepper, cut into strips
- 1 green bell pepper, cut into strips
- 2 cucumbers, sliced
- ½ cup balsamic vinegar
- 2 tablespoons olive oil
- 1 tablespoon sesame seeds, toasted
- 1 tablespoon basil, chopped

Directions:

1. In a bowl, combine the bell peppers with the cucumber and the rest of the ingredients except the sesame seeds and toss.
2. Sprinkle the sesame seeds, divide the mix between plates and serve as a side dish.

Nutrition Values:calories 226, fat 8.7, fiber 3.4, carbs 14.4, protein 5.6

27. Fennel and Walnuts Salad

Preparation time: 5 minutes

Cooking time: 0 minutes

Servings:4

Ingredients:

- 8 dates, pitted and sliced
- 2 fennel bulbs, sliced
- 2 tablespoons chives, chopped
- ½ cup walnuts, chopped
- 2 tablespoons lime juice
- 2 tablespoons olive oil
- Salt and black pepper to the taste

Directions:

1. In a salad bowl, combine the fennel with dates and the rest of the ingredients, toss, divide between plates and serve as a side salad.

Nutrition Values:calories 200, fat 7.6, fiber 2.4, carbs 14.5, protein 4.3

SOUPS AND STEWS

For more tips go to: Growthshape.com/health

28. White Bean Vegetable Soup

Servings 6

Preparation Time: 40 minutes

Ingredients:

- Garlic cloves - 2, chopped
- Carrots - 2, diced
- Olive oil - 2 tbsp.
- Shallots - 2, sliced
- Celery - 2 stalks, sliced
- Chicken stock - 4 cups
- Water - 2 cups
- Rosemary - 1 sprig
- White beans - 2 cans, drained
- Salt and pepper - to taste

Directions:

1. Pour olive oil in a pot and heat. Then add in garlic and shallots, cooking for approximately 5 minutes.
2. Mix in water, stock, rosemary, carrots, beans and celery and season with salt and pepper to suit your taste.
3. Cook an additional 15 minutes.
4. Serve up soup while fresh.

29. Chickpea Soup

Servings 8

Preparation Time: 45 minutes

Ingredients:

- Shallots - 2, chopped
- Garlic cloves - 6, chopped
- Olive oil - 3 tbsp.
- Celery - 1 stalk, diced
- Chickpeas - 2 cans, drained
- Chicken stock - 2 cups
- Water - 6 cups
- Dried oregano - ½ tsp.
- Carrots - 2, diced
- Dried basil - ½ tsp.
- Salt and pepper - to taste

Directions:

1. Heat oil and then add carrots, garlic, celery and shallots, cooking for 5 minutes.
2. Toss in chickpeas, basil, oregano. Next, add water and stock and salt and pepper to taste.
3. Continue cooking for 20 additional minutes.
4. Serve soup warm.

VEGETABLES

30. Walnuts Yogurt Dip

Preparation time: 5 minutes

Cooking time: 0 minutes

Servings:8

Ingredients:

- 3 garlic cloves, minced
- 2 cups Greek yogurt
- ¼ cup dill, chopped
- 1 tablespoon chives, chopped
- ¼ cup walnuts, chopped
- Salt and black pepper to the taste

Directions:

1. In a bowl, mix the garlic with the yogurt and the rest of the ingredients, whisk well, divide into small cups and serve as a party dip.

Nutrition Values:calories 200, fat 6.5, fiber 4.6, carbs 15.5, protein 8.4

31. Herbed Goat Cheese Dip

Preparation time: 5 minutes

Cooking time: 0 minutes

Servings:4

Ingredients:

- ¼ cup mixed parsley, chopped
- ¼ cup chives, chopped
- 8 ounces goat cheese, soft
- Salt and black pepper to the taste
- A drizzle of olive oil

Directions:

1. In your food processor mix the goat cheese with the parsley and the rest of the ingredients and pulse well.
2. Divide into small bowls and serve as a party dip.

Nutrition Values:calories 245, fat 11.3, fiber 4.5, carbs 8.9, protein 11.2

32. Scallions Dip

Preparation time: 5 minutes

Cooking time: 0 minutes

Servings:8

Ingredients:

- scallions, chopped

- 1 garlic clove, minced

- 3 tablespoons olive oil

- Salt and black pepper to the taste

- 1 tablespoon lemon juice

- 1 and ½ cups cream cheese, soft

- 2 ounces prosciutto, cooked and crumbled

Directions:

1. In a bowl, mix the scallions with the garlic and the rest of the ingredients except the prosciutto and whisk well.

2. Divide into bowls, sprinkle the prosciutto on top and serve as a party dip.

Nutrition Values:calories 144, fat 7.7, fiber 1.4, carbs 6.3, protein 5.5

33. Tomato Cream Cheese Spread

Preparation time: 5 minutes

Cooking time: 0 minutes

Servings:6

Ingredients:

- 12 ounces cream cheese, soft
- 1 big tomato, cubed
- ¼ cup homemade mayonnaise
- 2 garlic clove, minced
- 2 tablespoons red onion, chopped
- 2 tablespoons lime juice
- Salt and black pepper to the taste

Directions:

1. In your blender, mix the cream cheese with the tomato and the rest of the ingredients, pulse well, divide into small cups and serve cold.

Nutrition Values:calories 204, fat 6.7, fiber 1.4, carbs 7.3, protein 4.5

34. Pesto Dip

Preparation time: 5 minutes

Cooking time: 0 minutes

Servings:6

- Ingredients:
- 1 cup cream cheese, soft
- 3 tablespoons basil pesto
- Salt and black pepper to the taste
- 1 cup heavy cream
- 1 tablespoon chives, chopped

Directions:

1. In a bowl, mix the cream cheese with the pesto and the rest of the ingredients and whisk well.
2. Divide into small cups and serve as a party dip.

Nutrition Values:calories 230, fat 14.5, fiber 4.8, carbs 6.5, protein 5.4

SNACKS

For more tips go to: Growthshape.com/health

35. Tasty Beet Chips

Preparation time: 1 hour and 10 minutes

Cooking time: 30 minutes

Servings:4

Ingredients:

- 2 beets, sliced
- A pinch of sea salt

For the vinaigrette:

- 1/3 cup champagne vinegar
- A pinch of black pepper
- 1 cup olive oil
- 1 teaspoon green tea powder

Directions:

1. Put the vinegar in a small saucepan and heat over medium heat.
2. Add green tea powder, stir well, bring to a simmer, take off heat and leave aside to cool down completely.
3. Add the oil and a pinch of black pepper, whisk well and keep in the fridge for 1 hour.
4. Add beets slices and a pinch of salt, toss to coat well and arrange them on a lined baking sheet.
5. Place beet chips in the oven at 350 degrees F and bake for 30 minutes.

6. Leave them to cool down completely before serving them for your next party as a snack.

7. Nutrition Values:calories 100, fat 2, fiber 2, carbs 3, protein 2

36. Mediterranean Appetizer Salad

Preparation time: 10 minutes

Cooking time: 0 minutes

Servings:4

Ingredients:

- ½ cup black olives, pitted and sliced
- 3 zucchinis, cut with a spiralizer
- 1 cup cherry tomatoes, halved
- Salt and black pepper to taste
- 1 small red onion, chopped
- ½ cup canned chickpeas, drained
- ½ cup feta cheese, crumbled

For the mint tea vinaigrette:

- 1 tablespoon shallot, chopped
- ½ cup sunflower oil
- ½ cup olive oil
- ¼ cup apple cider vinegar
- 2 teaspoons mint tea powder
- 1 teaspoon mustard

Directions:

1. In a bowl, mix shallot with sunflower oil, olive oil, vinegar, mustard and mint tea powder and whisk well.
2. In a salad bowl, mix zucchini noodles with olives, tomatoes, onion, chickpeas, salt and pepper and stir gently.

3. Add the vinaigrette, toss to coat well and serve with the cheese on top.

Nutrition Values:calories 200, fat 3, fiber 2, carbs 4, protein 2

37. Greek Olives Spread

Preparation time: 10 minutes

Cooking time: 0 minutes

Servings:10

Ingredients:

- ounces hummus
- ½ cup kalamata olives, pitted and chopped
- 1 tablespoon Greek yogurt
- A pinch of salt and black pepper
- 1 avocado, pitted, peeled and chopped

Directions

1. In a blender, mix the hummus with olives, yogurt, avocado, salt and pepper, pulse well, divide into small cups and serve as an appetizer.

Nutrition Values:calories 130, fat 2, fiber 2, carbs 12, protein 5

38. Peppers Spread

Preparation time: 10 minutes

Cooking time: 0 minutes

Servings:6

Ingredients:

- 16 ounces canned chickpeas, drained
- ¼ cup Greek yogurt
- ounces roasted red peppers, minced
- Juice of 1 lemon
- 3 tablespoons tahini paste
- 1 tablespoon olive oil
- 3 garlic cloves, minced
- A pinch of salt and black pepper

Directions:

2. In a blender, mix the chickpeas with red peppers, the yogurt, lemon juice, tahini paste, oil, garlic, salt and pepper, pulse well, divide into small cups and serve as an appetizer.

3. Nutrition Values:calories 143, fat 8, fiber 3, carbs 15, protein 5

39. Warm Hummus and Lamb

Preparation time: 10 minutes

Cooking time: 5 minutes

Servings:16

Ingredients:

- 16 ounces chickpeas hummus
- 12 ounces lamb meat, ground
- A drizzle of olive oil
- ½ cup pomegranate seeds
- ¼ cup parsley, chopped
- A pinch of salt and black pepper

Directions:

1. Heat up a pan with the oil over medium-high heat, add the ground meat and brown for 5 minutes.
2. Spread the hummus on a platter, and then spread the lamb meat over it.
3. Sprinkle salt, pepper, pomegranate seeds and parsley all over and serve as an appetizer.

Nutrition Values:calories 154, fat 7, fiber 6, carbs 12, protein 6

40. Cucumber Cups with Red Pepper Hummus

Preparation time: 10 minutes

Cooking time: 0 minutes

Servings:20

Ingredients:

- 2 big cucumbers, cut into ½ inch thick slices and seeds scooped out
- 2 cups canned chickpeas, drained
- ounces canned red peppers, roasted, drained and chopped
- ¼ cup lemon juice
- 1/3 cup tahini paste
- 1 garlic clove, minced
- Salt and black pepper to taste
- ¼ teaspoon cumin, ground
- 3 tablespoons olive oil
- 1 tablespoon hot water

Directions:

1. In a food processor, mix red peppers with chickpeas, olive oil, tahini, lemon juice, salt, pepper, garlic, cumin and hot water and blend well.
2. Arrange cucumber cups on a platter, fill each with chickpeas mix and serve right away as an appetizer.
3. Nutrition Values:calories 182, fat 1, fiber 3, carbs 4, protein 2

41. Delicious White Bean Hummus

Servings:16/

Preparation time: 10 minutes

cooking time: 25 minutes

Ingredients:

- Roasted Tomatoes as needed
- 1 head of garlic
- 30 ounce cooked cannellini beans
- 1 tbsp lemon juice
- 1/2 tsp salt

Directions:

1. Set the oven to 400 degrees F and let it preheat meanwhile remove the tip of the garlic head and loose papery coating.
2. Get a 6 ounce custard cup and add garlic. Drizzle with 1 tsp of oil and then cover it with foil.
3. Place your custard into the heated oven and bake for 25 minutes until the garlic head is soft. When it is done uncover the custard cup let it cool and squeeze the garlic.
4. Place the garlic into a food processor and add the cannellini beans lemon juice oil and salt. Pulse until well blended.
5. Tip the hummus into the bowl and drizzle with olive oil. Add roasted tomatoes and serve with some vegetables.

SALADS

For more tips go to: Growthshape.com/health

42. Salad made with Avocado

Preparation Time: 10 minutes

Servings: 6

Ingredients:

- chopped fresh cilantro – ¼ cup
- peeled, pitted and diced avocado – 2
- pepper and salt to taste
- chopped sweet onion - 1
- large chopped ripe tomato - 1
- juiced lime – 1 2
- chopped green bell pepper – 1

Directions:

1. Add cilantro, avocados, tomato, onion, lime juice and bell pepper in a medium bowl together. Toss it until it is evenly coated in a gentle way. Add pepper and salt to taste.

43. Refreshing Zoodle Salad

Preparation Time: 20 minutes

Servings: 4

Ingredients:

- package arugula – 1 (5 ounce)
- small zucchini – 2
- fresh basil – 10 leaves
- cubed fresh mozzarella – 16 ounces
- balsamic vinaigrette – 2 tbsps or to taste
- grape tomatoes – 1 (10 ounce) basket

Directions:

2. Using spiralizer, cut into spirals zucchini (fitted with large shredding blade). Cut into smallest pieces zoodles.

3. In a bowl, add tomatoes, zoodle pieces, vinaigrette and mozzarella together and mix very well. Then refrigerate until it is ready to use.

4. Mix with basil and arugula before serving.

44. Jicama Salad

Preparation Time: 50 minutes

Servings: 6

Ingredients:

- Peeled navel oranges – 2 (cut into chunks)
- grounded black pepper to taste
- large red bell pepper - 1 (cut into bite-size pieces)
- juiced lemon - 1
- diced hothouse cucumber – 1 2
- thinly sliced radishes - 4
- chopped bunch cilantro – 1 2
- sliced small sweet yellow peppers – 3
- diced jalapeno pepper – ½
- sliced small sweet orange peppers - 2
- Minced Thai chile peppers - 3
- peeled and julienned large jicama - 1

Directions:

1. In a large bowl, combine Thai Chile peppers, red bell pepper, radishes, jicama, jalapeno pepper, black pepper, orange chunks, cucumber, lemon juice, sweet yellow and orange peppers, radishes, and cilantro.

2. Refrigerate after covering the bowl with plastic wrap and allow it flavors to blend, for 30 minutes.

45. InsalataCaprese recipe

Preparation Time: 15 minutes

Servings: 6

Ingredients:

- extra virgin olive oil – 3 tbsps
- large ripe tomatoes – 4 (sliced 1 4 inch thick)
- black pepper to taste (freshly grounded)
- fresh basil leaves – 1 3 cup
- fine sea salt to taste
- pound fresh mozzarella cheese - 1 (sliced 1 4 inch thick)

Directions:

1. In an overlap and alternate manner, arrange on a large platter mozzarella cheese slices, tomato slices and basil leaves.
2. Add seasoning sea salt and pepper after drizzling with olive oil.

46. Anchovy Dressing Romaine

Preparation Time: 10 minutes

Servings: 6

Ingredients:

- Parmesan cheese - ¼ pound
- Minced clove garlic – 1
- Pepper and salt to taste
- Rinsed and patted dry anchovy fillets – 2
- Extra virgin olive oil – ¼ cup
- Fresh lemon juice – 2 tsps
- Head romaine lettuce - 1

Directions:

1. Cut romaine leaves across into 1 2-inch-wide pieces after separation, wash well, and turn dry.
2. With a vegetable peeler, shave 1 3 glass parmesan twists in a blender anchovies and puree garlic with lemon juice.
3. With engine running include oil in a stream until dressing is emulsified. Season with salt and pepper.
4. In a bowl hurl romaine with dressing, 1 4 glass parmesan twists, and salt and pepper to taste. Partition serving of mixed greens between 2 plates and sprinkle with outstanding parmesan twists.

47. Orzo and Chicken Salad

Preparation Time: 1h1 minutes

Servings: 4

Ingredients:

- diced grilled chicken breast half - 1
- uncooked orzo pasta – ½ pound
- sprigs fresh oregano - 4
- olive oil – ¼ cup
- black olives – ¼ cup (cut in half lengthwise)
- red wine vinegar – 1 3 cup
- ground black pepper – ¼ tspn
- Dijon mustard – 1 tspn
- onion powder – ¾ tspn
- garlic powder – ¾ tspn
- dried basil – ¾ tspn
- salt – ½ tspn
- grape tomatoes – ½ cup (cut in half)
- crumbled feta cheese – 2 ounces
- red bell peppers – 2 (cut in half lengthwise and seeded)
- dried oregano – ¾ tspn

Directions:

1. In a big pot, fill with softly salted water and convey to a moving bubble over high warmth. When the water is bubbling, mix in the orzo, and come back to a bubble. Cook the pasta revealed, mixing at times, until the pasta has cooked through, yet is

still firm to the chomp, around 11 minutes. Channel well in a colander set in the sink, exchange to a bowl, and let cool in the fridge.

2. In a little bowl, whisk together the olive oil, red wine vinegar, Dijon mustard, garlic powder, oregano, basil, onion powder, salt, and pepper. In a huge bowl, blend together the cooked orzo, tomatoes, olives, feta cheddar, and chicken bosom meat until altogether consolidated. Pour the dressing over the orzo blend, softly blend to coat all fixings with dressing, and spoon into the red pepper parts. Enhancement each presenting with an oregano sprig.

DESSERT

For more tips go to: Growthshape.com/health

48. Crab Cake Recipe

Ingredients:

- Spice mix:

- Dried chili-1

- Comino seeds- 1 tsp

- Black peppercorns- 1 2tsp

- Fennel seeds- 1tsp

- Crab Cake:

- White crab meat(fresh or frozen)-8ozs. 250g

- Cooked potatoes (mashed)-8ozs. 250g

- Juice and grated zest of 1 2lime

- Medium sized onion (finely chopped)

- Chopped coriander- a handful

- Garlic- 1 clove(finely chopped)

- Salt

- Coating:

- Plain flour- 4 tbsps mixed with salt

- Olive oil

- Egg- 1 (beaten)

- Fresh white breadcrumbs- 4ozs 125g

Directions:

- Using an electric coffee grinder or a pestle and mortar, blend all the spices until it becomes a fine powder.

- Put all the Ingredients: in a mixing bowl and mix well until it becomes uniform.

- Make the mixture into cakes of your choice.

- Spread the flour in a plate, the beaten egg in a bowl and the breadcrumbs in another bowl.

- Coat each cake with flour and then dip into the egg and coat evenly then coat with breadcrumbs.

- Pour some olive oil in a nonstick fry pan and heat up, then gently cook the crab cakes on one side until it turns golden brown and turns over until the other side also turns golden brown.

- Serve immediately.

- Serving options: garnish with salad leaves, tomato salad on the side; you can also sprinkle some chopped coriander.

49. Salmon Escabeche

Ingredients:

- Salmon fillets- 2lbs. 900g
- Dry white wine- 10fl.ozs 1 2 a pint
- White wine vinegar- 10fl.ozs 1 2 a pint
- Soft brown sugar- 3tsps
- Garlic- 3 cloves(sliced)
- Carrot-1 (French cut- like match sticks)
- Olive oil-4ybsps
- Salt-2 Tsp
- Red bell pepper (small-sized)- 1 (French cut)
- Black peppercorns- 12
- Star anise- 2
- Onion(medium sized)- 1 (sliced)
- Coriander seeds-12
- Salt
- Pepper

Directions:

1. Season salmon fillets with salt and freshly ground black pepper, brown in olive oil and set aside.
2. Then add the remaining Ingredients: except for the wine, vinegar, and salt to frypan and fry until golden.
3. Add the wine, vinegar, sugar, and salt then boil till it is reduced by half.
4. Set the salmon fillets in a shallow dish and pour the marinade over and ensure that

the fillets are completely covered.

5. Cover with a plastic wrap and leave to cool.

6. Keep in the refrigerator overnight.

7. Enjoy your meal.

50. Seafood Risotto

Ingredients:

- Raw mussels-8 (debearded and raw)
- Small clams- 4ozs. 125g
- Whitefish (Hake, cod or similar)- 4ozs. (Cut into 5cm 2" pieces)
- Raw jumbo shrimps king prawns- 1 2kilo 1lb (shelled and deveined keep 4 aside for garnishing, save the heads for the stock)
- Stock (fish or vegetable stock)- 700mls
- Onion(medium-sized)- 1 (finely chopped)
- Round grain tice- 200g 7ozs
- Celery- 2 sticks(finely sliced)
- Extra virgin olive oil- 2-3 tbsp's
- Garlic- 2 cloves (bashed)
- Fresh dill- 1 tbsp (chopped)
- Dry white wine or vermouth- 1 glass (add to stock after cooking the fish, allow to stay warm but do not boil)
- Salt
- Freshly ground black pepper
- Parsley- handful (chopped)

Directions:

1. Pour stock into a medium-sized saucepan and allow to boil over on high heat.
2. Put all the fish into the pan and cook for 2 minutes only.
3. Remove the fish from the pan and keep in a covered bowl to keep warm.
4. Then add the prawn heads and allow to simmer for 5 minutes.

5. Remove prawn heads from stock and dispose of.

6. Add the dill then reduce the heat.

7. Then add the wine or vermouth; keep the stock under the boil but ensure it stays hot.

8. In a medium-sized heavy based pan, fry the onion and celery in the olive oil over medium heat until they become translucent.

9. Add the garlic and cook for another minute.

10. Add the rice and seasoning and cook for 2-3minutes stirring continuously until it becomes opaque.

11. Increase the heat to medium level.

12. Start adding the stock wine mixture little by little, a small portion at a time stirring continuously.

13. As the rice simmers down; it will reduce in size, then add another portion of the stock wine mixture.

14. Continue doing this and ensure that the risotto is well reduced before adding more liquid.

15. At this point, the rice mixture will start to look creamy as the rice cooks until all the liquid has been added. This takes about 15-20minutes.

16. Put in all the fish except the prawns with their shells and the mussels and mix gently.

17. Remove pan from the heather and cover it with its lid; then allow to cool for 3-4minures- this allows the flavors to seep into the rice and produces a creamier risotto.

18. Make sure the seasoning is adequate.

19. Serve immediately and garnish with the whole prawns and the mussels on the half shell.

20. Sprinkle parsley on top.

21. Serve immediately.

4 WEEK MEAL PLAN

DAY	BREAKFAST	LUNCH/DINNER	DESSERT
1	Sweet Potato Tart	Grapes, Cucumbers and Almonds Soup	Dorado – Baked Fish
2	Farro Salad	Spiced Eggplant Stew	Cod Recipe
3	Raspberries and Yogurt Smoothie	Pork and Rice Soup	Fish Pie Recipe
4	Blueberries Quinoa	Tomato, Sweet Potatoes and Olives Stew	Grilled Monkfish Recipe
5	Stuffed Pita Breads	Chicken, Carrots and Lentils Soup	Seafood Salad Recipe
6	Endives, Fennel and Orange Salad	Creamy Salmon Soup	Mackerel Recipe
7	Cranberry and Dates Squares	Baked Breaded Chicken	Seafood and Chicken Paella Recipe
8	Yogurt Figs Mix	Creamy Chicken Soup	The Lubina a la sal – Sea Bass
9	Tuna Sandwich	Buttered Garlic Shrimp	Sole Recipe
10	Tuna and Cheese Bake	Sautéed Pork Lettuce Cup Wraps	The Marinated Chicken
11	Seeds and Lentils Oats	Chicken and Beans Soup	Whole Fish
12	Lentils and Cheddar Frittata	Sage Pork and Beans Stew	The Poached Salmon
13	Cinnamon Apple and Lentils Porridge	Bread and Veggies Salad	The Grilled Shrimp
14	Coriander Mushroom Salad	Mint Chicken Soup	Fish Fillet
15	Salmon Frittata	Caraway Pork Stew	Crab Cake Recipe
16	Cottage Cheese and Berries Omelet	Parsley Beef Stew	The Mediterranean Tilapia
17	Potato and Pancetta Bowls	Marvellous Turkey Meatballs	Sardine Recipe
18	Cheesy Eggs Ramekins	Coriander Pork and Chickpeas Stew	Speedy Fat Bombs
19	Mango and Spinach Bowls	Delicious Chicken Goujons	Fluffy Chocolate Mousse with Strawberries

20	Veggie Salad	Mustard Chicken Thighs	Cashew Cakes
21	Bacon, Spinach and Tomato Sandwich	Cheesy Spinach Chicken Bake	Chocolate Pudding in a Mug
22	Eggs, Mint and Tomatoes	Turkey Soup with Zoodles	Mini Chocolate Cheesecakes
23	Baked Cauliflower Hash	Herbs Stuffed Roast Chicken	Hazelnut Truffles with Berry
24	Greek Beans Tortillas	Barley and Chicken Soup	Dark Chocolate Hazelnut Chocolate Bark
25	Tapioca Pudding	Potato Soup	KetoCreme Caramel
26	Apricots Couscous	Chili& Sage Flattened Chicken	Macadamia Ice Cream
27	Oregano Quinoa and Spinach Muffins	Mushrooms and Chicken Soup	Seafood Risotto
28	Salmon and Bulgur Salad	Beef and Cucumber Mix	Salmon Escabeche
29	Lettuce and Strawberry Salad	Pork and Lentils Soup	Cardamom Cookies
30	Herbed Quinoa and Asparagus	Baked Zucchini Stuffed with Shrimp & Dill	Anchovy Recipe